Anti-Inflammatory Slow Cooker Recipes

Gluten Free, Dairy Free, Soy Free and Nightshade Free

By Paula C. Henderson

Anti-Inflammatory Slow Cooker Recipes

Gluten Free, Dairy Free, Soy Free and Nightshade Free

ISBN: 9781712221914
Imprint: Independently published

Copyright © 2019 Paula C. Henderson. All Rights Reserved.

All rights reserved. No part of this book may be reproduced in any form or by any electronic or mechanical means including information storage and retrieval systems, without permission in writing from the author. The only exception is by a reviewer, who may quote short excerpts in a review.

Medical Disclaimer. ... The Content is **not** intended to be a substitute for professional **medical advice**, diagnosis, or treatment. Always seek the **advice** of your physician or other qualified health provider with any questions you may have regarding a **medical** condition.

Paula C. Henderson
Visit my website at www.Monumental-Ladies.us

Printed in the United States of America

First Printing: Nov 2019

ISBN: 9781712221914

Imprint: Independently published

Contents

THE ANTI-INFLAMMATORY DIET 8
BARBECUE SAUCES 13
    BBQ Sauce 1 13
    BBQ Sauce 2 14
    BBQ Sauce 3 15
    BBQ Sauce 4 16
    BBQ Sauce 5 16
    BBQ Sauce 6 16
BEANS 17
    Pinto Beans 19
    Refried Beans 20
BEVERAGES 21
    Apple Cider 22
BREAKFAST 23
    Bacon Jam 23
    Cinnamon & Brown Sugar Sweet Potato 24
    Fried Apples 25
    Overnight Oatmeal 26
FRUIT 27
    Poached Bosc Pears with Caramel Sauce 28
MEAT AND SEAFOOD 29
    Apricot Chicken with Kalamata Olives 29
    Asian Beefy Noodles 31
    Asian Lettuce Wraps 32
    Bacon Wrapped Pork Loin 33

Baked Ham	34
Balsamic Chicken	35
BBQ Pork Ribs	36
Beef and Broccoli	37
Beef Lettuce Wraps	38
Bolognese	39
Chicken and Mushrooms with Sauce	40
Chicken Pazole	41
Chicken Puttanesca	42
Chicken Tagine	43
Corned Beef and Cabbage	44
Glazed Ham	45
Indian Fish Curry	46
Kielbasa and Kraut	47
Lemon Garlic Chicken Breast	48
Lo Mein	49
Meatloaf	50
Peanut Chicken	51
Pesto Chicken Thighs	52
Poached Chicken Breast	53
Poached Salmon	54
Pork Chops and Apples	55
Pork Picnic Roast	56
Pork Roast with Onion Gravy	57
Saucy Meatballs	58
Savory Coconut Chicken	59

- Shredded Chicken 60
- Shrimp Scampi 61
- Sloppy Joes 62
- Smothered Pork Chops 63
- Steak Dinner 64
- Thai Meatballs 65
- Whole Chicken 67

RICE DISHES 68
- Artichokes, Spinach and Rice 68
- Chicken Broccoli and Rice 69
- Fried Rice 70
- Rice Pudding 71
- Yellow Squash and Rice 72

SOUP 73
- Beef Stew 73
- Beefy Cabbage Soup 74
- Bone Broth 75
- Carrot and Sweet Potato Soup 76
- Chicken and Rice Soup 77
- Chicken and Sweet Potato Soup 78
- Chili 79
- Coconut Curry Shrimp 80
- Cream of Celery Soup 81
- Cream of Chicken Soup 82
- Italian Sausage and Kale Soup 83
- Split Pea Soup 84

Turmeric Chicken Soup 85

White Chicken Chili 86

VEGETABLES 87

Artichokes 87

Asparagus 88

Baked Sweet Potatoes 89

Collard Greens with Ham Hock 89

Cooked Cabbage with Bacon 90

Garlic Mushrooms 91

Glazed Carrots 92

Green Beans 93

Spaghetti Squash 94

Spinach 95

Spinach and Artichokes 96

Sweet Potato Pie 97

Summer Squash 98

White Sweet Potato Casserole 99

Whole Cauliflower 100

Supporting Ingredients 101

Nightshade Free Taco Seasoning: 103

Pork Seasoning 104

THE ANTI-INFLAMMATORY DIET

The anti-inflammatory diet looks different for everybody except for these commonalities:

- Gluten free
- Dairy free

Many find they also feel better omitting soy, grains, legumes, cruciferous, and nightshades.

The recipes that follow do include some legumes but, I included some tips you might try if you feel comfortable reintroducing them into your diet temporarily by cooking specifically according to the instructions included here. If not, please simply omit those recipes.

If there is any food mentioned here that you have found causes you any problems just omit the ingredient, substitute the ingredient or move on to the next recipe.

For those of you that avoid cruciferous such as cauliflower, broccoli, cabbage and brussels sprouts: I have had many clients report to me that they can eat them cooked, but not raw and so some of the recipes do include these foods.

Foods that fight inflammation, such as turmeric are fighting an uphill battle if you are consuming more foods that cause inflammation. Inflammation fighting foods should be included in your diet but they will be more beneficial to you if you also avoid foods that cause inflammation. If you stubbed your toe and took an over the counter pain reliever it isn't going to be very effective if you keep stubbing your toe.

Fish is one the best anti-inflammatory foods you could choose to incorporate as a regular part of your diet. I like fish/seafood but I ate it only on occasion and never as a part of my regular weekly diet. I tried eating fish once a week. Soon I realized I was again, not including it in my weekly rotation.

I decided to try three times a week and yes, that was the point that my brain and my taste buds began to expect it to be included in my regular weekly meals. I would regularly "feel like I wanted fish". Of course to do this you really have to find recipes to support eating it 3 times a week.

There are many varieties of fish and seafood. My go to recipes are fish tacos and poached fish. It is quite easy to prepare fish in your crock pot and not feel you have to stand over it like you do when preparing it on the stove or heat up the kitchen (at least in the summer) by using the oven.

Dark Green Leafy vegetables is the most nutritious food, in my opinion, that one can consume and will fight inflammation in the body. I want to be sure to caution those who are sensitive to Vitamin K due to its possible interaction with blood thinners. Other than that dark green leafy vegetables are a low carb, easy to prepare cold and hot and can be used in a variety of dishes.

For those who poo-poo iceberg lettuce because it is "mostly water" I would like to remind everyone that water is highly recommended for the body. What's left are vitamins and minerals. The high water content in iceberg actually helps the body to absorb the vitamins and minerals that not only make up the lettuce, but also the other foods you are eating with the lettuce.

There are spices that you can include in your diet like cinnamon, turmeric, garlic, black pepper and more.

Sugar is known to cause inflammation. Even natural sugars you find in fruit. Fruit is otherwise a very, very healthy food and so my advice is to avoid all fruits during your elimination phase or any time you have started to experience symptoms while you figure out what might be causing your symptoms.

Artificial ingredients found in overly processed foods are known to cause a host of health problems. Almost all people report better overall health when omitting all overly processed foods from their diet.

Fresh? Canned? Frozen?

I feel my best if I eat only from the produce department, using supportive ingredients like seasoning, oils and vinegars to create variety.

For the sake of convenience in our very busy lives we are thankful for frozen vegetables as well as canned.

I do know some who are so very sensitive they must avoid all foods that have been canned. Most of us are not and this is something you will have to decide in your own diet.

Having said that, my opinion is that during the elimination phase it is best to stick to fresh and frozen and avoid all canned foods.

When you do begin to introduce canned foods back into your diet, if you do at all, be mindful to choose canned foods that limit the ingredients to less than three ingredients: such as green beans, water, or salt.

Avoid packaged foods that are "seasoned".

Eating healthy can be as simple or complicated as you wish it to be. Searing a chicken breast and heating up green beans is hardly cooking from scratch or loading those ingredients into a slow cooker with a bit of broth is quite simple too.

If you are new to an anti-inflammatory diet my advice is that during the first 3-6 months focus on foods that are "naturally" approved. For example, avoid foods where you are trying to find a cheese substitute, for now.

One of the most important things a person can embrace is being open to trying new foods or old foods prepared differently which seriously, becomes a whole new dish that you can love as much as you did other dishes you will need to leave behind.

Start a list of dishes you already know and love that do not include cheese or a bun, or potatoes. These foods should go on a different list: Banned Foods List

Be specific with your banned foods list. French fries, doughnuts and fast food hamburgers. Start your Banned Foods List and continue to add foods to it as they occur to you.

Approved Foods List:

Steak, roasted chicken, sweet potatoes, green beans. Perhaps there are some Asian dishes you like that would not include nightshades, gluten or dairy?

If you feel stuck, walk your grocery store and in each department do an inventory of all the foods you would be able to eat. Write them down. Viewing these foods will help you to realize how many foods there really are and dishes you can easily put together.

Make a few rules for yourself and stick to them.

1. Drink water with meals.

2. Decide that you will not include bread or desserts with your meals.
3. Place obvious foods like pastry and doughnuts, candy bars and cola on your Banned Foods List and stick to it.
4. If you consume a food with a label, read the label. When you begin to eat less and less processed foods this will not be so cumbersome because fresh and NOT overly processed foods have no ingredients list or the list is 3 or less ingredients. Not a long, long list.
5. Lastly, trust me when I tell you that omitting sugars and overly processed foods from your diet will help you to not overeat on a lot less food. Omitting overly processed foods completely from your diet will also stop sweet and salty cravings you may now be experiencing.

I have to enjoy pureed carrots in place of tomato sauce. It is definitely a much milder taste profile but once I had left all of the processed foods behind I found that I no longer longed for the strong tastes. I use to love Ranch Dressing from a bottle and could not imagine life without it and yet now it taste awful to me.

A quick tip about using pureed carrots: You easily buy fresh carrots, boil until quite tender, drain and add back a small amount of fresh water. Canned carrots, with the liquid works well if you are not opposed to canned vegetables. If you prefer to discard the liquid you can easily replace the liquid with fresh water. Frozen carrots are not suggested.

For a chili or taco flavor profile add Worcestershire sauce to the pureed carrots.

For an Italian sauce add balsamic vinegar to the pureed carrots.

BARBECUE SAUCES

Find your favorite gluten free, dairy free, soy free and nightshade free barbecue sauce for your chicken or pork and use as you normally would.

BBQ Sauce 1

- 1 tablespoon lemon juice
- 1 tablespoon apple cider vinegar
- ¼ cup pure maple syrup
- 1 tablespoon bacon fat
- 1 teaspoon ground ginger
- 1 cup canned, drained carrots. Pureed
- 1 cup minced onion
- 1 teaspoon salt

Optional: Black Pepper if you want some heat.

Using a saucepan, combine the syrup, lemon juice, vinegar, ginger, onions, carrots, salt and bacon fat. If you don't have bacon fat you could use ½ teaspoon of liquid smoke.

Bring to a boil. Turn the burner down and allow to simmer. Simmer about 20 minutes.

BBQ Sauce 2

- One 15oz can pumpkin
- 6 tablespoons apple cider vinegar
- 2 tablespoons cooking oil
- 2 tablespoons molasses
- 2/3 cup maple syrup or honey
- 6 smashed and minced garlic cloves or 1 teaspoon garlic powder
- 2 teaspoons salt
- 2 tablespoons Lea & Perrins Worcestershire Sauce (gluten free)
- 1/8 teaspoon ground ginger

Combine all ingredients in a saucepan and bring to a boil. Lower the heat to a simmer. Simmer about 15-20 minutes.

BBQ Sauce 3

- ¾ cup yellow mustard
- ¼ cup honey
- ¼ cup brown sugar
- 2 teaspoons Lea & Perrin Worcestershire Sauce (gluten free)
- 1 teaspoon garlic powder
- 1 teaspoon onion powder
- ½ teaspoon salt
- 1 teaspoon ground black pepper (more for more heat)

Combine all into a saucepan. Bring to a boil. Lower to a simmer and simmer for about 20 minutes.

BBQ Sauce 4

- 1 cup mayo
- ¼ cup white vinegar
- 2 teaspoons prepared horseradish
- ½ teaspoon salt
- ½ teaspoon black pepper
- ½ teaspoon garlic powder
- ½ teaspoon cumin

Combine in a saucepan. Heat to a light boil. Simmer about 10 minutes. This sauce is good hot or cold!

BBQ Sauce 5

- 1 cup grape jelly
- 1 cup prepared yellow mustard

Warm lightly in a saucepan and combine well.

BBQ Sauce 6

Molasses
Mustard

Warm lightly in a saucepan to combine very well.

BEANS

I wanted to include legumes to offer some variety and it gives me the opportunity to discuss why some people with arthritis avoid legumes because, for some, it causes painful inflammation.

What many, not all, but many of my clients have reported is that canned legumes cause them painful inflammation and so they avoid legumes in their regular diet. What we have found for many is that if legumes are prepared from dried beans, in a very specific way, many find that they can eat legumes without any painful issues.

You may want to try this method. Avoid canned legumes. Instead:

1. Buy a bag of dried beans.
2. Soak them overnight.
3. Drain, rinse well and then cook in your slow cooker or insta-pot.

Many find that skipping the instruction of soaking overnight (which I never did prior) can still experience pain. So do not skip any of the steps!

If legumes cause you problems simply omit them from your diet. Otherwise, legumes are gluten free, dairy free, soy free and nightshade free with the exception of soybeans. Here is a list of some of the most common legumes that are okay to include:

Adzuki beans	Lentils
Black beans	Lima beans
Chick peas	Navy beans
Fava Beans	Peanuts (yes, peanuts, but
Garbanzo beans	not all nuts, are legumes)
Green peas	Pinto beans
Kidney beans	Red beans

Pinto Beans

- One pound bag of pinto beans
- 1 garlic clove, smashed and minced
- 1 teaspoon salt
- 1 tablespoon oil
- 1 bay leaf
- water

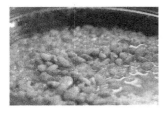 Soak the beans overnight. Next day, drain and rinse a couple of times. Transfer to the slow cooker. Add the garlic, salt, oil, and the bay leaf. Fill the slow cooker with water.

Cook on low 8 hours.

You could, of course, substitute many a legume for the pinto using this method: northern, navy, lima, butter bean, black bean, etc.

Just avoid soy or edamame bean if you are avoiding soy.

Refried Beans

- 1 onion, peeled and halved
- 3 c. dry pinto beans, rinsed
- 2 T. minced garlic
- 5 tsp. salt
- 2 tablespoons black pepper
- 1/8 tsp. cumin
- 1 1/2 tsp. fresh ground black pepper
- 9 c. water

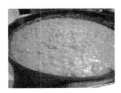

Soak the beans overnight. Drain and rinse twice.
Place the beans, onions, black pepper, garlic, salt, pepper, and cumin into a slow cooker.
Add 8-9 cups water.
Cover. Cook on low for 8 hours, or high for 4 hours. Adding more water as needed. The beans are done they should be very soft and tender.
Once the beans have cooked, strain the broth into a bowl, and reserve, as you will need it.
Using a handheld potato masher, mash the beans, adding the reserved water from slow cooker as needed to attain desired consistency. Taste and add salt and black pepper to taste.
Add 1-2 tablespoons of lime juice if desired. Stir well.

BEVERAGES

There are many gluten free, dairy free, soy free and nightshade free beverages to choose from:

Non-alcoholic Beverages:

- Water
- Tea
- Lemonade
- Sparkling Water
- Coffee
- Carbonated Beverages like cola and soda.
- Juice
- Kool-Aid
- Non-dairy milks, excluding soy milk:

Almond milk. If you are avoiding soy, please check "dairy-free" milk blends, yogurts, cheeses and butters as many of them include soy or soy byproducts.

Adult Beverages:

- Champagne
- Rum (plain unflavored rum only)
- Tequila
- Wine

Vodka is generally made from potatoes, a nightshade. Beer and whiskey are a gluten. Having said that there are many brands who have come out with gluten free beer and whiskey so feel free to check your local stores and be sure to read the label.

Remember that you can use coconut milk, bitters, and triple sec which are all gluten free, dairy free, soy free and nightshade free to make drinks.

Apple Cider

- 8 gala apples
- 4 cinnamon sticks
- 1 tablespoon whole cloves
- 1 tsp allspice
- 10 c water
- 1/2 c brown sugar

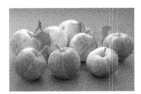

Wash, core and peel the apples. Place the apples in the slow cooker, add the cinnamon, cloves, allspice and all of the water. You will add the brown sugar later.
Cook on high 3-4 hours or low 6-8 hours.
Apples should be very, very soft and mushy.
Remove the apples with a slotted spoon, mash well and return to the slow cooker.
Add in brown sugar. Cook an additional 1-3 hours on low.
Combine well before straining the solids from the liquids.
Discard solids and store liquids in an airtight container for up to 1 week or freeze for later use.

BREAKFAST

Bacon Jam

- 1 pound sliced bacon, cut crosswise into 1-inch pieces
- 2 medium yellow onions, diced small
- 3 garlic cloves, smashed and peeled
- 1/2 cup apple cider vinegar
- 1/2 cup packed dark-brown sugar
- 1/4 cup maple syrup
- 3/4 cup brewed coffee (reg or decaf is fine)

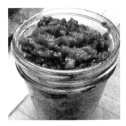

Fry the bacon in a skillet until cooked through and sort of crispy. Pour off all but 1 tablespoon fat from skillet; add onions and garlic, and sauté about 5 minutes. Add vinegar, brown sugar, maple syrup, and coffee and bring to a boil, stirring and scraping up browned bits from skillet. Add bacon and stir to combine.

Transfer mixture to slow cooker and cook on high, **uncovered**, until liquid is syrupy, 3 - 4 hours.
Remove from the slow cooker to a bowl and allow to cool about half hour minimum or longer. It just needs to be cooled off before putting into the food processor but not refrigerated cold. Transfer to a food processor; pulse until coarsely chopped. Let cool, then refrigerate in airtight containers, up to 4 weeks.

Cinnamon & Brown Sugar Sweet Potato

- Wrap each sweet potato individually in foil.
- Place in a dry slow cooker.

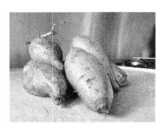

Cook on low about 6-8 hours overnight.
Top with your favorite dairy free butter, cinnamon and brown sugar. Raisins or sautéed apples optional.

Fried Apples

- 6 gala apples
- 2 tbsp cornstarch
- 1/4 cup granulated sugar
- 1/4 cup brown sugar
- 1 tsp cinnamon
- 1 tsp vanilla
- 1/4 cup non-dairy butter melted
- 1 tbsp lemon juice

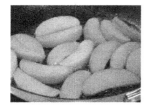

Spray the crockpot with a nonstick cooking spray
Turn crock pot on to high setting so it can be heating up while you gather your ingredients.
Peel, core and slice the apples and place in the crockpot
Toss the apples with 2 tbsp cornstarch until apples are coated well.
In a small bowl, combine granulated sugar, brown sugar and cinnamon.
Then, toss in with the apples.
For best results toss the apples with the cornstarch first. Mix the sugar and cinnamon in a small bowl first and then toss the cornstarch coated apples with the combined sugar and cinnamon.
Top apples melted butter, vanilla and lemon juice and stir to combine.
Cook on high for 2 hours or until apples are tender without falling apart.

Overnight Oatmeal

- 3 c. full fat canned coconut milk
- 2 c. water
- 2 c. gluten free old-fashioned oats
- 1/4 c. brown sugar
- 2 tbsp. maple syrup, plus more for serving
- 2 tsp. vanilla extract
- 2 tsp. cinnamon
- 1/4 tsp. salt
- 1 c. frozen blueberries

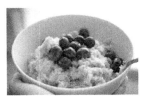

Spray the inside of the slow cooker with a non-stick cooking spray.
Add in all ingredients except the blueberries. Cook, stirring occasionally, on high for 4 hours, or on low for 8 hours.
In the last 10 minutes of cooking, turn dial to warm and gently stir in the blueberries.
Serve topped with maple syrup.

FRUIT

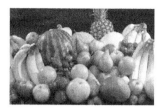

Here is a short list of some of the most popular fruits that are gluten free, dairy free, soy free and nightshade free.

- Apples
- Apricots
- Bananas
- Blackberries
- Blueberries
- Cantaloupe
- Grapefruit
- Kiwi
- Melon
- Oranges
- Papaya
- Pears
- Raspberries
- Strawberries
- Watermelon

Poached Bosc Pears with Caramel Sauce

- 1-1/2 cups brown sugar
- 1 Tbsp grated ginger root
- 3 Tbsp non-dairy butter
- 4 firm, slightly under ripe Bartlett or Bosc pears
- 1/8 tsp ground cinnamon, for garnish

In a skillet, stir together the sugar, ginger and butter and cook over low/med heat.

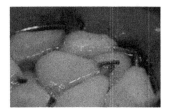

Peel the pears. Cut each pear in half lengthwise, and remove the stem and core.

Gently toss the pears with the sugar mixture. Pour the melted butter and sugar mixture into the slow cooker and layer the pears cut side down on top of the sauce.

Cook on high for 2 hours. One hour into cooking baste pears with sauce.

Remove the pears and set aside.

Pour the caramel sauce into a small sauce pan, bringing to a boil. Reduce the heat to low, to keep the sauce at a simmer. Shaking the pan fairly constantly, reduce the caramel sauce by about half of its original volume (don't let the caramel get too dark, or it will have a burnt taste). Should really only take about 3 minutes.

Place 1-2 pear halves per person on individual plates. Spoon a bit of sauce over the pears, and sprinkle with cinnamon. Serve warm.

MEAT AND SEAFOOD

Apricot Chicken with Kalamata Olives

- 2 pounds boneless, skinless chicken thighs
- 1 tablespoon oil
- 2 onions, cut into large chunks
- 4 cloves garlic, minced
- 1" piece ginger, peeled and minced
- 2 tablespoons chicken Broth
- 1 teaspoon salt
- ½ teaspoon turmeric
- 2 cups chopped parsnips
- 5 cups chopped butternut squash (about 1 small)
- ½ cup dried apricots, quartered
- ½ cup Kalamata olives, pitted
- ½ lemon, juice and zest reserved
- Cilantro and cooked rice, for serving

Turn the slow cooker to high.

Add the oil to a skillet. Sear the chicken thighs on both sides in the skillet. Not cooking through, just browning on both sides. Transfer to the slow cooker.

Add the onions to the skillet, and sauté, stirring, for about 5 minutes, or until lightly browned.

Add the garlic and ginger and cook, stirring, for 30 seconds, or until fragrant. Transfer to slow cooker.

Add the broth, salt, and turmeric to the slow cooker and stir to combine.

Add the root vegetables: squash, apricots, olives, lemon juice, and zest, and stir to combine.

Cook on low 6 hours or high 4 hours.

Use rice made yesterday or that has set at least an hour in the refrigerator. Reheat in the skillet tossing in finely chopped fresh cilantro or parsley. Rice for this dish is best when made using chicken broth instead of water. Also add 1 tablespoon oil, salt and pepper prior to cooking the rice. Cover and let it sit in the frig or on the counter for at least an hour.

Asian Beefy Noodles

- 2 T. extra virgin olive oil
- 1 T. apple cider vinegar
- 1 T. minced garlic
- 1 T. peeled and minced ginger root
- 1/2 C. coconut aminos
- 1/2 C. water
- 2 lbs. flank steak (sometimes called London Broil)
- 1/4 C. cornstarch
- 1 C. grated carrots
- 1 C. raw baby spinach
- 8 oz. baby bella mushrooms, sliced to 1/4"
- 1 teaspoon black pepper
- Salt if needed to taste
- Serve with gluten free spaghetti or go low carb spaghetti squash

Place first six ingredients in the slow cooker. Stir to combine.
Cut steak in half (lengthwise). Slice against the grain, 1/4" slices.
Toss sliced steak in cornstarch.
Put the meat in the slow cooker. Turn it in the sauce to coat. Cook on low for four hours.
Add carrots, spinach and mushrooms to the slow cooker and continue to cook another 30-60 minutes.
When the meat is done, tender, and mouth-watering, serve over zoodles, noodles or rice.

Asian Lettuce Wraps

- 1/4 cup coconut aminos
- 2 tablespoons rice vinegar
- 2 teaspoons sesame oil
- 1 tablespoon oil
- 2 pounds ground turkey
- 1 small bunch green onions — thinly sliced
- 1 tablespoon ginger
- 2 cloves garlic, smashed and minced
- 1 cup grated carrots
- 1 tablespoon black pepper
- 2 cans water chestnuts, drained and finely chopped, 8oz cans
- 2 heads butter or iceberg lettuce

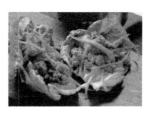

Spray slow cooker with nonstick spray. In a small bowl, stir together coconut aminos, rice vinegar, and sesame oil. Set aside.
Heat the oil in a large skillet over medium high. Add the ground turkey and brown the meat, breaking it into small pieces. Continue cooking until no longer pink, about 4 to 6 minutes. Stir in the green onions, ginger, and garlic. Cook 30 additional seconds.
Transfer the meat mixture to the slow cooker. Stir in the carrots, black pepper, and sauce you made using the coconut aminos, vinegar and sesame oil.
Cover and cook on LOW for 2 hours. Cooking on the low setting instead of the high setting is strongly suggested for best outcome. Stir in the water chestnuts and green parts of the green onions.
To serve, separate the butter lettuce leaves and fill with the chicken mixture. Enjoy hot.

Bacon Wrapped Pork Loin

- 3 pound pork loin , trimmed of excess fat
- 1 tablespoon oil
- 1 teaspoon salt
- 1 teaspoon pepper
- 4 garlic cloves , smashed and minced
- 1/3 cup brown sugar
- 8 slices bacon

Rub the pork loin with the oil, salt and pepper.

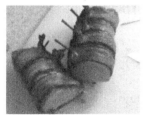

Rub the garlic and brown sugar to the top of the pork.
Wrap the pork with the bacon. Secure with water soaked toothpicks or short metal skewers.
Place into the slow cooker and cook on low for 4-5 hours.
If the bacon does not appear cooked or you would like to crisp it up when removed from the slow cooker, you can sear it in a hot skillet or place the pork loin on a baking sheet and place under the broiler for a few minutes on each side.

Baked Ham

- 1 Ham, pre-cooked, spiral cut - bone-in or boneless
- 3 1/2 cups brown sugar
- 1/2 cup Raw natural Honey
- One 20 oz can pineapple tidbits or chunks - do not drain

Place 2 cups of the brown sugar in the bottom of the slow cooker.
Add the ham next.

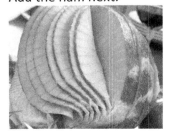

Spread the honey over the ham allowing it to make it's way into the cut spirals.
Place the pineapple around the sides, including the juice.
Spread the remaining brown sugar to the top of the ham.

Cook on low for about 4 hours.

Balsamic Chicken

- 3 boneless skinless chicken breast
- 1/2 cup balsamic vinegar
- 1/2 cup chicken broth
- 1/4 cup brown sugar
- 3 cloves garlic, minced
- 1 teaspoon dried basil
- 1/2 teaspoon dried oregano
- 1/4 teaspoon dried thyme
- 1/2 teaspoon salt
- 1/2 teaspoon pepper

Combine vinegar, broth, sugar and garlic in a bowl; set aside. Season chicken breasts with basil, oregano, thyme, salt and pepper.

Place chicken breasts into a slow cooker. Stir in balsamic vinegar mixture. Cover and cook on low heat for 7-8 hours or high for 3-4 hours

BBQ Pork Ribs

- 3 lbs country style pork ribs
- oil
- salt
- 1 1/2 cups grape jelly
- 12 oz yellow mustard
- 1 tbsp black pepper (optional for heat)

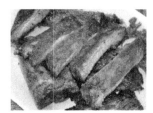

Rub oil and salt over all sides of the ribs.
In a separate bowl combine jelly and mustard well. Add black pepper if you want some heat or, you can also add horseradish.
Toss the ribs with the sauce, add to the slow cooker.
Cover and cook on low for 7-8 hours, or until tender.

Beef and Broccoli

- 2 lbs. sirloin steak, sliced thin
- 1 cup beef broth
- ½ cup coconut aminos (an alternative to soy sauce)
- ¼ cup brown sugar
- 1 Tablespoon sesame oil
- 3 garlic cloves, minced
- 4 Tablespoons cornstarch
- 4 Tablespoons water
- 1 (12 oz.) bag frozen broccoli florets
- White rice, cooked

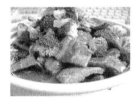

Whisk together beef broth, coconut aminos, brown sugar, sesame oil, and garlic.
Place sliced beef in the liquid and toss to coat in the slow cooker. Cover with lid and cook on low heat for 5 hours.
When done, whisk together cornstarch and water in small bowl. Pour into crock pot and stir to mix well. Add the frozen broccoli over the beef and sauce. Gently stir to combine. Cover with lid and cook 30 minutes to cook broccoli and thicken sauce.

Beef Lettuce Wraps

- 2 pounds sirloin steak, thin slices
- 4 cloves garlic, smashed and minced
- 1/4 cup coconut aminos
- 1 tablespoon honey
- 1 tablespoon rice vinegar
- 1 tablespoon sesame oil
- 1 tablespoon sesame seeds
- 1 teaspoon ground ginger

Garnish: thinly sliced scallions

Place beef in crockpot.
Mix remaining ingredients in a medium bowl and pour over beef.
Cook on low setting for 6-8 hours.
Spoon into lettuce cups with your favorite toppings, wrap, and enjoy! You could also serve with rice or gluten free spaghetti

Bolognese

- 1 pound ground beef
- 1/2 cup red wine
- 1 cup) chicken stock
- 1 tsp dried oregano
- 1/2 tsp thyme
- 1 tsp basil
- 1/2 cup) onion, finely diced
- 2 tbsp worcestershire sauce
- 2 large carrot, finely diced
- 2 tsp corn starch
- Season with salt & pepper

When dicing up the carrots and onion, keep the size uniform. Preferably about the size of a pea. I use an electric food chopper!

In a skillet over medium high heat brown the ground beef.

Add the cornstarch, stir around to coat well.

Add the red wine and simmer on high for 1 minute (this burns off the alcohol).

Add prepared ground beef and wine to slow cooker along with chicken stock, onion, carrot, worcestershire, oregano, basil, and thyme.

Cook on high about 2 hours, stirring often if possible! Or, you can cook on low 4 hours, stir well, turning the slow cooker to high for about 30 minutes before tossing with gluten free spaghetti.

Chicken and Mushrooms with Sauce

- 4 boneless chicken breasts
- 2 cups fresh sliced mushrooms
- 1 small onion, chopped
- 2 garlic cloves
- 1/5 cups chicken broth
- 2 tablespoons corn starch
- Salt and pepper

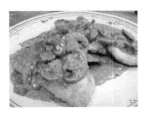

Sear the chicken in a hot, oiled skillet before adding to the slow cooker.
Add the chicken and the remaining ingredients, except the corn starch, to the slow cooker.
Cook on low 4-6 hours depending on the size of your chicken.
When the chicken is cooked through remove and set aside.
Mix corn starch and a few spoonful's of the broth to form a smooth paste. Add the paste, slowly while whisking, back into the slow cooker.
Return the chicken, cover, turn on high and let cook another 30 minutes.

Chicken Pazole

- 4 cups chicken broth
- 3 boneless skinless chicken breasts
- 1 white onion, chopped
- 2 cloves garlic, minced
- 2 tbsp. cumin
- 1 teaspoon coriander
- 1 tbsp. oregano
- 2 tsp. kosher salt
- Freshly ground black pepper
- 2 c. (15-oz.) cans hominy, drained
- Thinly sliced radishes
- Thinly sliced green cabbage
- Fresh cilantro, chopped

Place broth, chicken, onion, garlic, cumin, coriander, oregano, salt and pepper into the slow cooker. Cook on low for 6 to 8 hours, until the chicken is tender and cooked through.

Take chicken out of slow cooker and shred with two forks. Return to the slow cooker along with the hominy and cook for another 30 minutes.

Serve soup into bowls and garnish with radish, cabbage and cilantro.

Chicken Puttanesca

- 4 chicken thighs bone in and skin on
- 1 medium onion diced
- 4 cloves garlic, smashed and minced
- 3 tablespoons oil
- 1/2 cup chicken broth
- Two 15 ounce can of carrots with the liquid
- 1 teaspoon Italian seasoning
- 1 tablespoon capers
- 1/2 cup olives, sliced (remove the pimento which is a nightshade)
- 3 tablespoons balsamic vinegar
- 2 tablespoons cornstarch
- salt and pepper to taste (heavy on the black pepper if you want more heat)

Rub chicken with oil, and then with salt and pepper on all sides. Brown the chicken on both sides in a hot skillet and then set aside. Just brown. Do not cook through.
Sprinkle the cornstarch on the chicken (in the skillet) and toss around to coat the cornstarch.
Puree the carrots and liquid in a blender until smooth. Set aside. Stir in broth and deglaze the pan. Scrape the browned bits off the bottom. Stir in pureed carrots, Italian seasoning, balsamic vinegar, capers and olives.

Add all ingredients to the slow cooker. Cook on low 4-6 hours to cook chicken through and allow everything to marry.

Chicken Tagine

- 6 chicken thighs, skin-on and bone-in
- 4 tablespoons cornstarch
- 1 medium red onion, halved, then sliced 1/4 inch thick
- 1/4 cup oil

- 1 teaspoon ground cinnamon
- 1 teaspoon ground ginger
- 1/2 teaspoon turmeric
- 1/2 teaspoon black pepper
- 1 1/4 teaspoons salt
- 4 garlic cloves, finely chopped
- 5 fresh cilantro, finely chopped
- 5 sprigs fresh flat-leaf parsley, finely chopped
- 1 1/2 cups chicken broth
- 2 tablespoons honey
- 1/2 cup dried apricots, separated into halves
- 1/3 cup whole blanched almonds

Combine the seasonings and the cornstarch in a bowl. Toss the chicken in the seasoning to coat well. Heat the oil in a large pan over a medium heat. Add the chicken and sear both sides to a golden brown. Place in slow cooker.
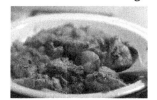
Using the same skillet, sauté the onion just until softened. Add the chicken and onion to the slow cooker.

Add the remaining ingredients, the honey, the parsley, cilantro, apricots and broth to the slow cooker.

Cook on Low 5 hours until the chicken is cooked through. Stir very well before serving.

Garnish with the flaked almonds and serve with rice.

Corned Beef and Cabbage

- 1 corned beef brisket (2-3 lbs)
- 1 medium yellow onion, cut into large wedges
- 3 large carrots, cut into thirds
- 2 stalks celery, cut into thirds
- 1 large or two medium sweet potatoes, peeled and quartered (white sweet potatoes or orange)
- 1 teaspoon salt
- 1 teaspoon black pepper
- 1 packed pickling spice
- 1/2 teaspoon thyme
- 2 bay leaves
- 1/2 green cabbage, cut into large wedges

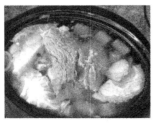

Place potatoes, carrots, celery and the onion in the crock pot.
Put the corned beef on top of the vegetables and be sure to season generously with salt, pepper, & pickling spices.
Add bay leaves and fill crockpot with water until just below the top of the meat.
Cook on high for 5 hours, until meat is tender. Add cabbage to the top (do not combine) and cook on high another 45 minutes to 1 hour more until cabbage is tender and cooked through. Remove meat and vegetables from slow cooker, slice and serve. Optionally, you could steam the cabbage in a steamer on the stove and serve with the prepared corned beef.

Glazed Ham

- 1 cup brown sugar
- 1/3 cup honey
- 1/4 c. Dijon mustard (make your own Dijon by combining yellow mustard and horseradish)
- 1/2 tsp. garlic powder
- 1/2 teaspoon salt
- 1/2 teaspoon black pepper
- 1 cup pineapple juice
- 1 (4-6 lb.) spiral cut ham

Combine sugar, honey, juice, mustard, and garlic powder in a medium sauce pan and season with salt and pepper. Whisk ingredients together and bring to a simmer.
Cook until reduced slightly, about 5-7 minutes.
Place ham in slow cooker and separate slices slightly.
Pour glaze over ham. Cook on low about 6 hours.
Baste every hour.
Serve with the glaze on the side.

Indian Fish Curry

- 1/3 cup oil
- 1.5 cups chicken broth
- 1 yellow onion, diced
- 2 garlic cloves, smashed and minced
- 1-inch piece fresh ginger, peeled and grated
- 2 tablespoons cornstarch
- 1 tablespoon ground cumin
- 2 teaspoon ground coriander
- 2 teaspoon brown mustard seeds
- 2 teaspoon ground turmeric
- 1 can carrots, pureed with liquid
- 1 tablespoon balsamic vinegar
- 1 tablespoon sugar
- salt and black pepper
- 2 lb. white fish fillets such as cod or halibut, cut into 1-inch chunks
- 3 tablespoon chopped fresh cilantro

Sauté the onion and cook, stirring, until it begins to turn golden, 5 minutes in a skillet. Stir in the garlic, ginger, cumin, coriander, mustard and turmeric and the cornstarch. Stir to coat all vegetables well and cornstarch "disappears".
Pour in 1 1/2 cups broth into the skillet scraping up the browned bits on the bottom and transfer to slow cooker.
Add the pureed carrots, sugar, and balsamic vinegar to the slow cooker. Cook on low for 2 hours. Check the sauce halfway through the total cooking time; if it seems to be getting too thick, stir in more water, about 1/2 cup at a time.
Uncover and add the fish, stirring gently to coat it with the sauce. Re-cover and continue to cook on low for about 30 minutes more. Taste and adjust salt and pepper.
Serve with cooked rice and top with fresh chopped cilantro or parsley.

Kielbasa and Kraut

- 1/2 cup dairy free butter
- 1 medium onion, diced
- 2 garlic cloves, minced (four if you are a garlic lover)
- 1/2 teaspoon thyme leaves
- 1/4 teaspoon ground sage
- ground black pepper, to taste
- 3 **white** sweet potatoes, peeled and diced
- 1 (16 ounce) can or bag sauerkraut
- 1 lb beef kielbasa, cut into bite size slices

Combine all ingredients in the slow cooker.
Cook on low 6 hours or high 3 hours or until the potatoes are tender.

Lemon Garlic Chicken Breast

- 2 pounds boneless chicken breasts
- 1 teaspoon oregano
- ½ teaspoon salt
- ¼ teaspoon black pepper
- 2 tablespoons dairy free butter or cooking oil
- ¼ cup water
- 3 tablespoons lemon juice
- 2 garlic cloves, mashed and minced

Combine the oregano, salt and pepper and rub all of each of the chicken breasts.
Heat oil or butter in a skillet and sear both sides of the chicken until golden brown.
Place the chicken in the slow cooker.
Add the water, lemon juice, and garlic.

Cook on low about 6 hours.

Lo Mein

- 2 pounds boneless pork shoulder
- 3 cups broccoli florets
- 2 carrots, julienned
- 2 stalks celery, diced
- 1 cup snow peas
- 1 (5-ounce) can sliced water chestnuts, drained
- 1 pound gluten free spaghetti

FOR THE SAUCE
- 1/3 cup coconut aminos (a soy sauce alternative)
- 3 cloves garlic, minced
- 2 tablespoon brown sugar, packed
- 1 tablespoon Worcestershire Sauce (Lea & Perrins is a gluten free brand)
- 1 tablespoon oyster sauce
- 1 tablespoon freshly grated ginger
- 1 teaspoon sesame oil

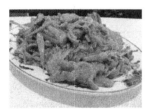

Combine together coconut amino, garlic, brown sugar, Worcestershire, oyster sauce, ginger and sesame oil in the slow cooker.
Add pork shoulder.
Cook on low heat for 8 hours.
REMOVE pork shoulder from the slow cooker and shred the meat before returning to the pot with the juices. Stir in broccoli, carrots, celery, snow peas and chestnuts. Cover and cook on high heat for 15-30 minutes, or until vegetables are tender.
COOK pasta according to package instructions; drain well.
SERVE pasta immediately, topped with pork mixture.

Meatloaf

- 1 lb. 80%-93% lean ground beef (that has never been frozen) For best results choose the ground beef in the Styrofoam try, not the tube.
- ½ cup dried bread crumbs (toast gluten free sandwich bread or purchase premade gluten free bread crumbs)
- 1/2 cup diced yellow onion
- 4 tablespoons minced celery
- 1/2 cup chicken, beef, mushroom or vegetable broth
- 1 large egg beaten
- 2 tbsp. Worcestershire sauce
- 3/4 tsp. salt (increase salt to 1 teaspoon if you are adding the mushrooms)
- 1/4 tsp. ground black pepper
- Optional: add 1/4 cup minced baby portabella mushrooms (this adds moisture and a nice flavor profile)

Combine all ingredients very well. I find it best to beat the egg in a separate bowl before adding to the meat mixture.

Pat into a loaf.

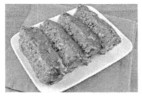

Cook on low in the slow cooker for 6 hours.
Allow to rest at least 15 minutes before slicing.

If you are looking for a ketchup like topping choose one of the BBQ Sauce recipes at the beginning of this book. Another quick topping is to mix ¼ cup molasses, honey, or brown sugar with ¼ cup prepared yellow mustard. Taste and adjust the mustard or molasses to your liking. I will sometimes add a pinch of horseradish or minced white onions.

Peanut Chicken

- 2 cloves garlic minced
- 2/3 cup peanut butter
- 1 cup chicken broth
- 1 lb boneless skinless chicken breasts, cut into 1 inch cubes
- 1 cup thinly sliced zucchini (very thinly)
- 1/3 cup coconut aminos
- 1 tablespoon honey
- 1 tbsp lime juice
- 1 cup chopped cilantro divided
- chopped peanuts for garnish
- Gluten free spaghetti

Place all of the ingredients, except the pasta in the slow cooker. Stir to combine.

Cook on low for 4 hours or on high for 3 hours.
Just before serving add in lime juice and 1/2 cup of cilantro.

Serve over noodles and garnish with remaining cilantro and peanuts.

Pesto Chicken Thighs

- 3 lb boneless skinless chicken thighs
- 1/2 teaspoon salt
- 1/4 teaspoon pepper
- 1 jar (6.25 oz) basil pesto
- 2 tablespoons chicken broth
- 4 slices crispy crumbled bacon

Spray slow cooker lightly with cooking spray. Sprinkle chicken thighs with salt and pepper on both sides.
Brown both sides of the thighs in an oiled, hot skillet. Transfer to slow cooker.
Add pesto and broth to the skillet and scrape the bottom. Pour over chicken thighs, and spread evenly with spoon.
3 Cover and cook on High heat setting 4 hours. Top with crispy crumbled bacon when you serve.

To make homemade dairy free pesto:

2 packed cups basil leaves
1/2 cup olive oil (or more, depending on consistency you want)
1/2 cup roasted, unsalted pine nuts (or pecans, almonds or walnuts!)
3 cloves of garlic
1/2 teaspoon salt

Storing in the refrigerator: to help pesto from turning brown after you place the pesto in a mason jar. Pour a thick layer of olive oil on top. Leave this oil on the top, do not combine.

Poached Chicken Breast

- 2 bone-in, skin-on Chicken Breasts
- Oil, salt and pepper
- ½ cup water (the water should cover the bottom of you slow cooker and just halfway up the side of the chicken)

Rub the chicken with the oil, salt and pepper on all sides.
Spray the crock pot with non-stick cooking spray
Place the chicken and the water in the crock-pot

Cook on low 6 hours.

Poached Salmon

- 1-2 lb. salmon fillet
- Oil
- salt
- black pepper
- 1 lemon, cut into rounds
- 1 1/2 cup chicken broth
- Juice of 1/2 lemon

Line slow cooker with parchment paper. Add a layer of lemon slices to the bottom of the slow cooker.

Rub oil, salt and pepper on all sides of salmon and place top of the sliced lemon.

Add broth and lemon juice to slow cooker. Liquid should come only halfway up your filet.

Squeeze the juice of 1/2 a lemon over top of salmon. Cook on low 2 hours.

Pork Chops and Apples

- 4-6 boneless pork chops
- 3 apples sliced (such as Granny Smith)
- 1 medium onion sliced
- salt and pepper to taste

Rub each pork chop on both sides with salt and pepper.
Place pork chops in bottom of the slow cooker.
Add sliced apple and onions on top of pork chops.
Place lid on and let cook on low for 8 hours.

Pork Picnic Roast

- One 5lb boneless pork picnic roast
- 3 tablespoons oil
- 2 teaspoons salt
- 2 teaspoons black pepper
- 1 smashed garlic clove
- 1 pound fresh, raw baby carrots
- 1-2 stalks of celery
- 1 medium onion, chopped
- 1 cup beef broth

Optional: 1 fresh sweet potato chopped to bite size pieces or One 16oz fresh white button mushrooms, sliced in half.

Combine the oil, salt and pepper. Rub well all over the roast. Sear the roast in a hot skillet just until golden brown on all sides. Just about 3-5 minutes per side.
Place the roast in the bottom of the slow cooker.
Add the vegetables.
Add the broth and the garlic.

Cook on low 6-8 hours. If the roast is tough even though it is cooked through, it just needs to cook longer. The heat breaks down the toughness. How long you need to cook is dependent on the size of your roast.

Pork Roast with Onion Gravy

- 1 large onion
- 1/4 cup water or chicken broth
- 4–5 lb. pork roast (boston butt or pork shoulder)
- 2 Tbsp oil
- 2 garlic cloves, smashed and minced
- 2 tsp. black pepper
- 2 tsp. salt
- 2 tsp. dried thyme
- 2 tsp. dried rosemary
- 3 tablespoons cornstarch

Chop the onion and place in the slow cooker.
Pour water or broth in the slow cooker.
Combine the oil, garlic and spices together in a small bowl. Rub this mixture over all sides of the roast.
Place roast on top, so the fat side is up.
Cook on low 8-10 hours, until meat can be shredded with fork.
Remove the roast and one small bowl of the broth. Whisk in 3 tablespoons cornstarch and whisk until very smooth. Whisk into the still very hot broth. Cover and allow to cook while the roast rests.
Serve the pork shredded, with gravy on top.

Saucy Meatballs

- 1 pound ground beef that has never been frozen
- 4 tablespoons minced onion
- 1 whole egg
- 1 teaspoon salt
- 1 teaspoon black pepper
- 1 cup BBQ Sauce 5 from this book

Combine the ground beef, salt, pepper, egg and minced onion.
Form small golf ball size meatballs.
Brown all sides of each meatball in a hot skillet.

Add the meatballs and the BBQ sauce to the slow cooker. Cook on low about 4 hours.

Savory Coconut Chicken

- 2 pounds boneless skinless chicken breast, cut into bite size pieces
- One 15 ounce can coconut milk
- 1 can carrots, pureed with the liquid
- 2 tablespoons lemon juice
- 2 tablespoons cooking oil
- 1 yellow onion, chopped
- 5 garlic cloves, mashed and minced
- 3 teaspoons turmeric
- ¼ teaspoon ground ginger
- 3 tablespoons cumin
- 1 teaspoon black pepper
- 1.5 teaspoons salt
- 2 tablespoons gluten free Worcestershire sauce
- ¼ cup chopped fresh cilantro or parsley

Using the oil, sauté the onion and garlic (start with a cold pan), until soft. Add the ginger, turmeric, cumin, salt, and pepper. Cook another 2 minutes.

Transfer the onions, garlic and seasonings to your slow cooker. Add the chicken, coconut milk, pureed can of carrots, and lemon juice.

Cook on low about 6 hours.

Serve with fresh chopped cilantro over rice, cauliflower rice or gluten free pasta. Or, eat it like the sauce is a soup.

Shredded Chicken

- 3 pounds boneless skinless chicken breasts (fresh or frozen*)
- 1 teaspoon salt
- 1/2 teaspoon pepper
- 1/2 cup chicken broth if using thawed chicken. Omit if using frozen.

Combine all of the ingredients in the slow cooker.
Cook on high for 3 1/2-4 hours or on low for 5 hours.
Remove the chicken and shred chicken with two forks or with your hands using kitchen gloves.
Return shredded chicken to the slow cooker and cook for an additional 30 minutes on low. This step helps to keep the chicken moist and tender.

Shrimp Scampi

- 1/4 cup chicken broth
- 2 tablespoons oil
- 2 tablespoons non-dairy butter
- 1 tablespoon minced garlic
- 2 tablespoons finely chopped fresh parsley (an electric food chopper does a nice job)
- 1/2 freshly squeezed lemon
- salt and pepper to taste
- 1 pound raw shrimp, peeled & deveined (but leave tail on while cooking)
- Gluten free pasta

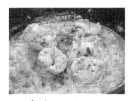

Place broth, oil, butter, garlic, parsley, lemon juice and salt and pepper in the slow cooker.
Stir in the shrimp.
Cook on high for 1 1/2 hours or on low for 2 1/2 hours.
About 10 minutes before shrimp is done boil the gluten free pasta in salt water. For best results use a large stock pot. Pasta cooks best in way more water than it seems you really need. Be sure the water is well salted and do not add the pasta until the water is at a full boil. Follow the timing instructions on your box of pasta.
Combine the cooked spaghetti with the shrimp and sauce before serving.

Sloppy Joes

Use a gluten free bun!

- 2 pounds ground beef
- 1 tablespoon cornstarch
- Two 15 ounce canned carrots
- ¼ cup minced celery
- 3 tablespoons gluten free Worcestershire sauce
- ½ teaspoon salt
- ½ teaspoon pepper (use more if you want a bit of heat)
- 1 teaspoon cumin
- ½ teaspoon garlic powder
- ½ teaspoon onion powder
- ¼ teaspoon liquid smoke

Brown ground beef in a skillet. Add all of the seasonings and the Worcestershire to the ground beef while browning in the skillet. Halfway through browning the ground beef add the minced celery.
Sprinkle everything in the skillet with the cornstarch. Stir around to coat well.
While the ground beef is browning, puree the carrots with the liquid in a blender until smooth.
Add all of the ingredients: the ground beef mixture, the pureed carrots and the liquid smoke to the slow cooker. Mix well.
Cook on high 2 hours or low 3-4 hours.

Smothered Pork Chops

- 4 bone-in average thickness pork chops (not the thin pork chops)
- 1/2 teaspoon pepper
- 1/4 teaspoon salt
- 4 slices bacon, cut into bite size pieces
- 1 large yellow onion, rough chopped
- 2 garlic cloves, smashed and minced
- 2 cups chicken broth
- 2 teaspoons Worcestershire sauce (GF)
- 1 bay leaf
- 4 tablespoons cornstarch
- 1 tablespoon cider vinegar
- 1 tablespoon prepared yellow mustard

Spray slow cooker with non-cooking spray. Pat pork chops dry with paper towels; season both sides with pepper and salt. Set aside.

In a skillet, fry bacon until crispy.
Keeping the skillet hot, now sear the pork chops until just browned, not cooked through. Add the onions and do a quick sauté just to soften.
In a small bowl, combine cornstarch and a few tablespoons of the broth until quite smooth. Add to slow cooker.
Add remaining broth, mustard, Worcestershire sauce, vinegar, garlic and bay leaves. Whisk ingredients in slow cooker to combine.
Put the bacon and the onions in the slow cooker.
Put the pork chops into slow cooker leaning the pork chops up against sides of slow cooker, bone side on the bottom.
Cover; cook on Low 2 hours.

Steak Dinner

- 2 ribeye steaks
- oil
- salt and pepper
- garlic cloves
- 3-4 white sweet potatoes
- 1 pound of fresh asparagus

Spray slow cooker with nonstick cooking spray.
Rub each steak with oil, salt and pepper on both sides. Place in the bottom of the slow cooker.
Pour 1/2 cup to 1 cup of your favorite steak sauce over the steaks. A1 is gluten free. Or, you could use beef or mushroom stock, or even Coconut Aminos for a soy sauce flavor.
Take a sheet of foil and top over the steaks
Spritz the top with either cooking oil or Pam
Cut 3 or 4 white sweet potatoes into thick medallions. Toss with oil, salt, pepper.
Place the white sweet potatoes medallions on the foil in the slow cooker. Add another layer of foil to completely cover the potatoes. Add your favorite vegetable to the top. You could use fresh asparagus (toss with oil, salt and pepper first)
You could add fresh green beans. Blanch the green beans, then toss with oil, salt and pepper. Whether using asparagus or green beans I like to add a couple of fresh garlic cloves, smashed and minced, to the top of the vegetable.
Option: Instead of potatoes and a green vegetable try onions in place of the potatoes and sliced mushrooms in place of the green vegetable. Be sure to follow the instruction of tossing with oil, salt and pepper before adding to the slow cooker.
Put your slow cooker lid on, turn it on low and cook about 6-7 hours.

The texture of your steak will be very tender, more like that of a roast, but without buying a roast!

Thai Meatballs

- 4 stalks lemongrass, roughly chopped
- 3 medium shallots, roughly chopped
- 6 medium cloves garlic
- 1 tablespoon black pepper
- 1 (3-inch) knob fresh ginger, peeled and cut into 1/2-inch pieces
- 3 tablespoons Asian fish sauce
- 2 teaspoons oil
- 1 cup sweet sauce (see recipe below)
- 2/3 cup light brown sugar
- 2/3 cup coconut aminos
- 1/2 cup rice vinegar
- 1 cup water
- 2 pounds ground turkey (choose ground turkey in the Styrofoam tray, not a tube)
- 1 cup gluten free bread crumbs, plus more if necessary
- 1 large egg
- 1/2 cup thinly sliced scallion, white and light green parts only, divided
- 1 teaspoon salt, more to taste
- 1/4 cup chopped cilantro leaves and tender stems
- 1/2 cup chopped unsalted peanuts
- 2 tablespoons fresh juice from 1 lime

Make the sweet sauce:

- 1/2 cup rice vinegar
- 1/2 cup brown sugar
- 2 teaspoons fresh ginger root, minced
- 1 teaspoon smashed and minced garlic
- 1 teaspoon cumin
- 1 can sliced carrots, pureed with the liquid
- 1 tablespoon black pepper
- 1 tablespoon Worcestershire sauce

- 1 tablespoon cornstarch

Pour pureed carrots and vinegar into a saucepan, and bring to a boil over med/high heat.
Stir in sugar, ginger, garlic, pepper, Worcestershire, cumin and cornstarch.
Mix very well while keeping at a boil 3-5 minutes. Remove saucepan from stove and set aside.

Ginger paste:
In the bowl of a food processor, combine lemongrass, shallot, garlic, ginger, and fish sauce.
Process until the mixture forms a paste.

Heat oil in a large skillet over medium heat. Add half of the ginger paste, reserving the rest for the meatballs.
Cook, stirring, about 2 minutes. Stir in sweet sauce and cook for 1 minute.
Stir in water and bring to a boil, stirring constantly. Reduce to a simmer and cook, stirring occasionally, until reduced by half.
Transfer the mixture to a slow cooker.

In a large bowl, combine reserved ginger paste with ground turkey, gluten free bread crumbs, egg, and half of the sliced scallion. Season with salt and pepper. Make golf ball sized meatballs.
Brown the meatballs on all sides in a skillet.
Add meatballs to slow cooker. Stirring to coat.
Cook on low 6 hours, or on high 3 hours.

In a small bowl, combine remaining scallion, cilantro, chopped peanuts, and lime juice.

Once the cooking time is up, switch the slow cooker to the "warm" setting. Right before serving, sprinkle approximately 3/4 of the peanut mixture over the meatballs and stir. Top with the remaining peanut mixture and serve.

Whole Chicken

- 2 tablespoons packed brown sugar
- 2 teaspoons cumin
- 1/2 teaspoon onion powder
- 2 teaspoons salt
- 1 whole chicken (3 to 4 lb)

1 Spray slow cooker with cooking spray.
2 In small bowl, stir together brown sugar, cumin, onion powder and salt.
3 Pat chicken dry, both inside and outside, with paper towels. Rub chicken all over with brown sugar mixture.
4 Place chicken, breast-side up, in slow cooker.
5 Cook on High 3 hours or until legs move easily when lifted or twisted and thermometer inserted in thickest part of inside thigh reads at least 165°F. Remove chicken from slow cooker; let rest 10 minutes before serving.

RICE DISHES

Artichokes, Spinach and Rice

- 1 cup long grain rice
- 1 can artichoke hearts, drained
- ½ cup frozen chopped spinach
- 2 garlic cloves, smashed and minced
- 1 tablespoon oil
- 1 teaspoon salt
- 1 cup chicken stock

Add all of the ingredients to the slow cooker. Cook on high for 2 hours or until the rice is done.

Chicken Broccoli and Rice

- 2 lbs boneless skinless chicken breast cut into 1-inch pieces
- 2 cups long-cooking white rice
- 1 1/2 cups unsweetened coconut milk
- 1 1/4 cups chicken broth
- 1 lime for juice and zest
- 1 tsp garlic powder
- 2 cups fresh or frozen broccoli chopped, bite size. If you use frozen broccoli use it straight from the freezer and only use 1 cup of water instead of 1 1/4 cup water.
- 2-3 green onions sliced
- salt and pepper to taste
- non stick cooking spray

Using a strainer, rinse the rice several times. Drain very well.
Spray the inside of the slow cooker to prevent sticking.
Put the rice, milk and broth in the slow cooker.
Add half the lime juice, garlic and half of the chopped green onion.
Put a layer of chopped fresh broccoli or frozen chopped broccoli on top of the rice.
Then a layer of fresh chopped chicken (raw) on top of the broccoli.
Now add the remaining lime juice and green onion.
Cook on high about 2.5 hours or until the rice is cooked.

Fried Rice

- 2 cups uncooked LONG grain rice
- 12 ounce bag frozen peas, carrots and corn
- 2 garlic cloves, smashed and minced
- 4 cups chicken broth
- 1/4 cup coconut aminos
- 1 teaspoon salt
- 3 tablespoons toasted sesame oil
- 2 large eggs, lightly beaten with fork
- 4 green onions, sliced

Add rice, then the frozen vegetables and garlic to the slow cooker.

In a bowl, stir together the chicken broth, coconut aminos, salt and sesame oil. Pour it over the vegetables.
Cook on HIGH for 2 hours.
Pour beaten eggs over the vegetables, close the lid and let it cook for another 45 minutes.
Stir the mixture, fluffing the rice with a fork.
Stir in the green onions.

Rice Pudding

- non-dairy butter
- 7 cups coconut milk, plus more as needed (from the carton)
- 2 cups long-grain white rice
- 3/4 cup sugar
- 1/4 teaspoon salt
- 1 cup raisins
- 2 tablespoons brown sugar
- 1/2 teaspoon cinnamon
- 1/2 teaspoon vanilla extract

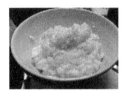

Rub the inside of the slow cooker with non-dairy butter.
Add 6 cups of the milk, all of the rice, sugar, and salt.
Combine well.
Cook on high until the rice is cooked through and the pudding is creamy, about 4-6 hours.
Stir in the remaining cup of milk, raisins (if using), brown sugar, cinnamon, and vanilla. Add additional milk as needed to reach the desired consistency. Serve immediately.

Yellow Squash and Rice

- 2 tablespoons olive oil
- 4 yellow squashes (8 ounces each), thinly sliced
- 2 garlic cloves, smashed and minced
- 1/2 cup chicken broth
- 1/4 cup long grain long cooking rice (it's all you'll need)
- Coarse salt and ground pepper

Add all of the ingredients to your slow cooker. Cover and cook on low about 6 hours or high about 4 or until the rice is cooked tender.

This is a wonderful dish, as is, when experiencing an upset stomach. You can easily dress this up with leftover meatloaf crumbled in, shredded cooked chicken or even leftover ham that has been cubed or cut into bite size pieces. If you are serving the basic recipe to guests top with crumbled crisp bacon.

SOUP

Beef Stew

- 2 tablespoons olive oil
- 2 pounds stew meat, cut into 1-inch cubes
- salt and pepper, to taste
- 2 sweet potatoes, peeled and chopped into bite size pieces
- 1 onion, diced
- 3 cloves garlic, minced
- 3 cups beef broth
- 2 tablespoon Worcestershire sauce
- 1 teaspoon dried thyme
- 1 teaspoon dried rosemary
- 2 teaspoon cumin
- 1/8 teaspoon coriander
- 2 bay leaves
- 3 tablespoons cornstarch

Heat olive oil in a large skillet over medium heat.
Season beef with salt and pepper, to taste. Sear the beef in the skillet on all sides. We are not cooking the meat through, just browning the outside. Sprinkle the beef with cornstarch and stir to coat all of the cornstarch. Place beef, potatoes, carrots, onion and garlic into a 6-qt slow cooker. Stir in beef broth, Worcestershire, thyme, rosemary, cumin, coriander and bay leaves until well combined; season with salt and pepper, to taste. Cover and cook on low heat for 7-8 hours or high heat for 3-4 hours or until beef is tender.

Tip: When cooking beef or pork in a crockpot or oven: even when the meat is cooked through by appearance and temperature, if it is tough, continue to cook the meat on high another hour for a more tender meat.

Beefy Cabbage Soup

- 1 pound ground beef
- ½ onion, chopped
- 1 medium head cabbage, chopped
- 2 stalks celery, chopped
- 1 carrot, chopped
- 2 cloves garlic, minced
- 5 cups beef broth
- 1 cup cooked kidney beans
- 1 tablespoon Italian seasoning
- 1 teaspoon salt

Brown ground beef in skillet.
Add the onion to the beef and continue cooking until meat is completely cooked through.
Drain the fat. Add ground beef and onion to slow cooker.
Add the celery, carrot, garlic, cabbage, beef broth, beans, Italian seasoning, and salt to the crockpot and cover.
Cook on high for 4 hours.

Bone Broth

Any broth you make from any bones is bone broth. This is an example using chicken bones but you can easily replace it with fish bones or beef or pork bones. I do not suggest mixing bones.

I like a pure stock/broth. This is how you make that. I find this to be more versatile later when using in a recipe. I also think it takes much better.

The trick here to get a rich stock is to first fill the crock pot with bones (save them in the freezer until you have enough or buy a bag of chicken wings) and then fill it full with cold water.

If the bones are left over from a hen, a roast, ribs, or other meat that has been cooked, you most likely will not have scum that rises to the top that will need skimmed off.

- 2 pounds chicken wings, necks, backs, or other parts (raw parts or carcasses from a rotisserie chicken or roast chicken)
- Cold water

Place the bones and water in your slow cooker, add enough cold water to cover completely. Cook on low for at least 12 hours or overnight. Skim the surface after the first 2 hours to remove any scum that floats to the top.
2. Strain and let cool completely.

Carrot and Sweet Potato Soup

- 1 pound carrots
- 1/2 lb sweet potatoes, orange
- 1/2 red onion, sliced
- 1 1/2 tsp Real salt, add more to taste
- 1 TB avocado oil
- 4 cups chicken stock
- 12 oz coconut milk (if you are not a fan you can use more broth instead, or a different non-dairy milk)
- 1 lime, zested and juiced
- 2" knob of fresh ginger, peeled and grated
- 1/4 tsp cinnamon or cumin
- 1/8 tsp ground cloves
- 1/8 tsp ground ginger
- a pinch of mace

Peel and chop carrots and sweet potatoes. Boil until quite tender.

In a blender or food processor puree the somewhat cooled off carrots and potatoes with the coconut milk. Add broth and continue to blend. Do this in batches if your blender or food processor is not large enough: half the carrots and potatoes with milk and or broth until all is pureed smooth.

Add the puree to the slow cooker.

Add lime zest and juice, fresh ginger, and seasonings to the slow cooker. If you have broth leftover and you want a thinner consistency use a whisk to blend it into the puree in the slow cooker.

Add all of the remaining seasonings.

Cook on low 3 hours. If you want an even silkier soup, push the soup through a mesh strainer before serving.

Chicken and Rice Soup

- 1 tablespoon oil
- 1 onion minced
- 3 large carrots peeled and diced
- 1 rib celery diced
- 1 teaspoon minced garlic
- 1 teaspoon dried parsley
- 1/2 teaspoon dried thyme
- 1/2 teaspoon sage
- 5 cups chicken broth
- 2 chicken breasts raw, cut into bite size pieces
- 3/4 cup long grain brown rice
- 1 teaspoon salt
- 1/8 teaspoon black pepper
- 1 tablespoon cornstarch
- 1 tablespoon apple cider vinegar

Spray slow cooker with a nonstick cooking spray. Add oil.
Turn slow cooker to high.
Toss chicken with cornstarch. Add to the hot slow cooker. Stir around to dissolve the cornstarch.
Add the remaining ingredients. Add the carrots last.
Cook on high 2.5 hours or until the rice and chicken are cooked.

Chicken and Sweet Potato Soup

- 3 med to large chicken breast, cut into bit size pieces
- 1 large sweet potato, peeled and chopped into bite size pieces
- 2 cups fresh kale, stems removed and chopped
- 6-8 cups sodium free chicken broth
- 3 teaspoons salt
- 2 teaspoons Italian seasoning
- 1 bay leaf

Place all of the ingredients in your crockpot. Cook on low about 6 hours.

Chili

- 1 pound ground beef
- 1 can carrots
- 1 can kidney beans
- ¼ cup gluten free Worcestershire sauce
- 1 T. apple cider vinegar
- 2 tablespoons cumin
- 1 tablespoons beef bouillon or use beef broth instead of water
- ¼ cup thinly sliced celery
- 1 medium onion, chopped
- 2 tablespoons corn starch
- 4 cups water or beef broth
- 2 tablespoons black pepper
- 1 teaspoon salt or more to taste

Brown the ground beef in a skillet. Sprinkle with cornstarch and stir around to coat.

Pour the can of carrots, with the liquid into your blender. Blend until pureed and smooth.

Add the ground beef, the pureed carrots, and all of the other ingredients to your slow cooker.

Cook on low 2-4 hours.

Coconut Curry Shrimp

Prep:
- 1 large white onion (roasted in oven)
- 1 bunch of scallions (green onions)
- 4 large heads of garlic (roasted in oven)
- 1 6-inch piece of fresh ginger (roasted in oven)

Wrap each ingredient (the onion, the scallions, the garlic and the ginger) in its own foil and bake in a 400 degree oven for 30 minutes or until soft.

Transfer to food processor, add a tablespoon of salt and puree until just smooth but do not over blend.

- 30 ounces coconut milk
- 15 ounces chicken broth
- 1/4 cup cilantro
- 1 ½ tsp cumin
- 1 tablespoon turmeric
- 1 tablespoon black pepper
- ½ tsp ground ginger
- 2 teaspoons coriander
- 1/4 cup packed cilantro leaves and stems
- 1 lb shrimp

Add coconut milk, broth, all of the seasonings, the roasted pureed ingredients and half of the cilantro to slow cooker. Stir to mix well.

Cook high 2 hours or low for 4 hours.

Add shrimp and cook an additional 10-30 minutes or until shrimp are done. Cook time for the shrimp depends on the shrimp size and your slow cooker. I suggest you check it every 10 minutes. Some find it is cooked through in the first 10 minutes, while others report that it takes 20-30 minutes. Garnish with remaining cilantro.

Cream of Celery Soup

- 1/2 cup Chopped Onion
- 3 cups chopped celery
- 1 peeled and cubed white sweet potato OR One 15oz can northern beans, pureed with liquid
- 1 teaspoon salt
- 2 cups chicken broth
- 1/2 teaspoon thyme
- 1 tablespoon black pepper
- 1/2 teaspoon garlic powder
- 2 tablespoons corn starch
- 1 tablespoon yellow mustard (prepared mustard)

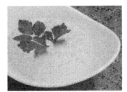

Add the chopped onion, celery, potato or pureed white beans to the crockpot. Add the chicken broth, salt, thyme, garlic powder, mustard, and pepper. Mix it and set the crockpot on low for 4 hours. After 4 hours, open the lid carefully and using a potato masher, mash all the celery mix. Or, remove half the soup with half the broth, allow to cool about 20 minutes and then puree in a blender or food processor. Return to slow cooker. Combine well. If the soup seems too thin, Mix the cornstarch and a couple tablespoons of water, and add this to the crockpot soup mix. Turn the slow cooker to high for 30 minutes or until hot.

Cream of Chicken Soup

- 5 tablespoons unsalted butter
- 5 level tablespoons cornstarch
- 4-6 cup chicken stock
- 2 garlic cloves, smashed and minced
- 3 tablespoons minced onion
- 1 teaspoon salt
- 1 teaspoon black pepper
- 1 cup shredded or bite size chopped **cooked** chicken
- 1/2 cup frozen peas and carrots
- 1 teaspoon apple cider vinegar
- Optional: sliced, sautéed mushrooms

Tip: be sure to use a good quality rich chicken stock or make a good strong, rich homemade stock of your own.

Melt the butter over medium low heat.
Whisk in the cornstarch
Gradually whisk in the chicken stock. Should thicken to the consistency of a creamy soup, not a gravy. Just add more stock if too thick.
Transfer the soup to the slow cooker. Add the remaining ingredients.
Cook on high 3 hours.

Italian Sausage and Kale Soup

- 1 lb ground pork (in the Styrofoam tray in the meat dept)(or use 4 turkey sausages instead of making your own, casings removed)
- 1 tablespoon fennel
- 1 tsp garlic powder
- 1 teaspoon salt
- 1 teaspoon black pepper
- 1 tbsp olive oil
- 4 cloves garlic minced
- 2 yellow onions, diced
- 1 large fresh carrot, chopped
- 2 stalks celery, chopped
- 1 tbsp Italian seasoning
- 4 cups chicken broth
- 1 (20oz) canned carrots
- 1 can chickpeas, drained and rinsed
- 2 cups kale, cut from stem and finely chopped
- 3 tablespoon gluten free Worcestershire sauce

Combine the ground pork with fennel, garlic powder, salt, black pepper and a tablespoon of oil.
Puree the can of carrots, with the liquid, in your blender until smooth.
Brown the pork mixture in a skillet.

Spray the slow cooker with a nonstick cooking spray. Add the pork and pureed carrots to the slow cooker.
Add the remaining vegetables and garlic, broth, drained chickpeas and Worcestershire sauce to the slow cooker.
Stir in the kale.
Cook on high for 3 hours.

Split Pea Soup

- (16 ounce) package dried split peas, rinsed
- 2 cups diced ham or a ham hock
- 3 carrots, peeled and sliced
- 1 medium onion, chopped
- 2 stalks celery, chopped
- 2 garlic cloves, smashed and minced
- 1 bay leaf
- 1/2 teaspoon salt
- 1/2 teaspoon black pepper
- 1 1/2 quarts chicken broth

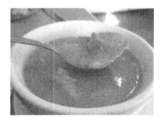

Layer ingredients in crockpot.
Pour in broth.
Cover and cook on high 4-5 hours or on low for 8 hours.
Remove Bay leaf.

Turmeric Chicken Soup

- 2 tbsp oil
- 1 medium onion, diced
- 3 celery stalks, chopped
- 2 medium golden beets, peeled and chopped
- 4 carrots, peeled and sliced
- 2 cups cauliflower, chopped
- 5 cups chicken stock
- 1 cup coconut cream (optional.. sub more bone broth)
- 10–12 oz chicken, cooked and shredded or boneless, skinless raw chicken cut into bite size pieces (will cook in slow cooker)
- 1.5 cups kale, destemmed and roughly chopped
- 2–3 tsp ground turmeric
- 1 tsp ground ginger
- 1/2 tsp black pepper
- Sea salt to taste
- 1/4 cup fresh parsley (plus extra for garnish)

Place all of the ingredients in the slow cooker.
If you are not a fan of coconut milk you simply replace that with one cup of chicken stock.
Cook on high 3 hours or until the chicken is cooked if using raw chicken OR cook on low 6 hours.

White Chicken Chili

- 1.5 pounds boneless skinless chicken breasts
- 4 cups chicken stock
- 2 cans white beans — (15-ounce cans) such as white kidney beans, cannellini, or Great Northern beans, rinsed and drained
- 1 cup thinly sliced celery
- 3 garlic cloves, smashed and minced
- 1 small yellow onion, diced
- 1 tablespoon apple cider vinegar
- 2 teaspoons ground cumin
- 1/2 teaspoon ground ginger
- 1 teaspoon dried oregano
- 1/2 teaspoon salt - more to taste
- 1 tablespoon black pepper
- 1/4 cup chopped fresh cilantro
- 3 tablespoons cornstarch
- Fresh lime wedges
- Avocado for topping

Cut raw chicken into bite size pieces or use cooked shredded chicken. Toss chicken with cornstarch and place in slow cooker. Add white beans, celery, garlic, onion, cumin, oregano, ginger, salt, black pepper and vinegar. Add any remaining cornstarch and stir to combine.

Add the broth.

Cover and cook on low for 4 to 6 hours or high for 2 to 4 hours, until the chicken is cooked through.

Squeeze lime juice into chili just before serving or place a lime wedge with each serving. This is wonderful topped with fresh ripe avocado or make a quick guacamole.

VEGETABLES

Artichokes

- 2-4 fresh artichokes, depending on the size of your crockpot. A wide crockpot, rather than a tall narrow crockpot is needed for each artichoke to sit firmly on the bottom of the crockpot.
- salt
- pepper
- 2 garlic cloves minced
- 1/2 lemon
- 1/4 cup dairy free butter, or Avocado Oil works well here.
- 1 cup water

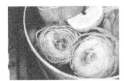

Cut the bottoms off the artichokes so they sit flat.
Cut about a half inch from the tops of the artichokes.
Spray the inside of the slow cooker with non-stick cooking spray.
Place the artichokes in the slow cooker.
Be sure each artichoke has room to sit flat on the bottom of your crockpot. You can remove a few of the outer leaves if needed to allow for this.
Sprinkle each artichoke with salt and pepper, then add a little garlic to the top of each artichoke.
Squeeze lemon juice over each artichoke.
Place a 1/2 teaspoon of butter, or a drizzle of oil on top of the artichokes.
Add the water to the bottom of the slow cooker.
Cook on HIGH for 4 hours.
Serve with melted butter or mayo

How Do You Eat a Fresh Artichoke?

The California Artichoke Advisory Board has a video on their web site showing you exactly how to eat a fresh, steamed artichoke. It is a short video but be sure to watch it to the end to see how to remove the artichoke heart.

>Here is the link: http://artichokes.org/how-to-eat

Asparagus

- 2 lbs fresh asparagus

Sauce:
- 5 tablespoons lemon juice
- 1/2 cup chicken broth
- 2 garlic cloves, smashed and minced
- 1 tsp salt
- 1/2 tsp black pepper

Place asparagus in the slow cooker.

Mix the sauce ingredients in a separate bowl before adding to the slow cooker.
Pour sauce over asparagus.
Cook on low 4 hours, or 2 hours on high.

Baked Sweet Potatoes

- Wrap each potato with foil individually.
- Cook in the slow cooker on high about 4 hours or low about 6 hours. Cooking time will depend on the size of each potato.

During the cold winter months I occasionally like to have a sweet potato with cinnamon and brown sugar for breakfast. On those occasions I put the potato in the crock pot before I go to bed and it's ready in the morning!

Collard Greens with Ham Hock

- 2 lbs collard greens washed & cut
- 2 large smoked ham hocks
- 1 large yellow onion chopped
- 1 tablespoon smashed and minced garlic
- 1 teaspoon salt
- 1 tablespoon black pepper
- 1 tablespoon oil
- 4 cups chicken broth
- 1 cup water
- 2 tbsp apple cider vinegar

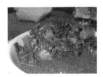

Place the ham hocks, onions, garlic, oil, salt and pepper into the slow cooker.
Add the broth.
Cook on high for 6 hours.
After 4 hours the ham hocks should be tender and falling off of the bone.
Add in the collard greens. Stir around.
Cook for another two hours. Stir in the vinegar just before removing from the slow cooker.

Cooked Cabbage with Bacon

- 1 small head of cabbage- cored and chopped
- 8 slices cooked crisp and chopped bacon
- 1 cup fresh chopped onions
- 8 cups chicken broth
- ¼ cup dairy free butter
- salt and pepper

Fry bacon until crisp, set aside to cool.
Sauté chopped onion slightly in the bacon fat.
Combine the chopped cabbage, sautéed onion and the crumbled bacon in slow cooker.
Top with remaining ingredients: the broth, dairy free butter, salt and butter.
Cover and cook on high for 4 -6 hours or until cabbage is tender.

Garlic Mushrooms

- One pound fresh whole mushrooms
- 4 garlic cloves, smashed and minced
- Oil
- Salt and pepper

Go ahead and place the mushrooms in the slow cooker. Toss well with oil, garlic, salt and pepper until well coated.
Cook on low about 3-4 hours or until tender.

If you want a sauce or gravy toss the mushrooms with cornstarch *AFTER* the oil, garlic, salt and pepper. Be sure the cornstarch is coated well.
Add 1 cup chicken or beef stock to the crock pot. Stir around, then cook.

Glazed Carrots

- 2 lbs carrots peeled and sliced into bite size pieces
- 1/4 cup non-dairy butter, melted
- 1/3 cup brown sugar
- 1/2 teaspoon salt
- 1/4 teaspoon cinnamon
- 1/8 teaspoon nutmeg
- 1 teaspoon cornstarch

In a small bowl, whisk together the butter, brown sugar, salt, cinnamon, nutmeg and cornstarch. Toss with carrots to coat. Transfer to slow cooker.
Cook on HIGH for 3 hours or until carrots are tender.

Green Beans

- 2 pounds fresh green beans, washed and trimmed
- 4 cups chicken broth
- 2 garlic cloves, smashed and minced
- 2 tablespoons minced onion
- 1 teaspoon salt
- 1 teaspoon pepper

Add all of the ingredients to the slow cooker. Cook on high about 4 hours or on low for 8 hours.

Spaghetti Squash

- A whole, fresh spaghetti squash that will fit in your slow cooker.
- ½ cup water

Using a paring knife, cut several slits into all sides of the squash.

Place the squash and the water in the slow cooker.

Cook on low 6 hours or until a knife easily goes through the rind.

Remove and allow to cool enough to handle. Slice the squash in half. Using an ice cream scoop remove the seeds. Removing the spaghetti squash from the shell can be done by using a fork. I like to turn the cut half over and merely peel off the softened rind. Then, using a fork, separate the squash into strands.

Spinach

- Turn your slow cooker to high, add ½ cup water and put the lid on.
- Toss fresh spinach with oil, salt and pepper.
- Add to slow cooker. Put the lid on and allow to cook on high for 30 minutes. Leave completely alone during the cook time. Remove, toss with a smidgen of balsamic vinegar and serve.

You can also use this method of cooking spinach if you have another food in the bottom of the slow cooker. For example if you are poaching chicken then you could add the spinach in this way to the top (do not combine, just lay on top) for the last 30 minutes of cook time.

Spinach and Artichokes

- 1 bag fresh spinach
- 1 can artichoke hearts, drained
- ½ cup chicken broth
- 2 garlic cloves, smashed and minced
- 1 teaspoon salt
- ½ teaspoon pepper
- 1 tablespoon oil
- 1 pound fresh mushrooms, sliced and sautéed (optional)

Combine all ingredients except the spinach in the slow cooker.
Add the spinach to the top without combining.
Cook on high 1 full hour.

Sweet Potato Pie

- 3 pounds sweet potatoes, peeled and chopped into bite size pieces
- 4 tbsp. melted dairy free butter
- 1 cups packed brown sugar
- 1/4 c. water
- 1 tsp. ground cinnamon
- 1/2 tsp vanilla
- 1/8 tsp salt
- 1 1/2 cup marshmallows
- 1/2 cup pecans

Spray Crock-Pot with cooking spray and add sweet potatoes. In a medium bowl, combine butter, sugar, water, cinnamon, vanilla, and a pinch of salt. Whisk to combine. Pour over sweet potatoes and toss until they are fully coated. Cook on high for 4 hours, stirring often.

Remove lid and top with marshmallows and pecans. Reduce heat to low and cover. Cook on high about 10 minutes more or until marshmallows are melted.

Summer Squash

- 2 tablespoons oil
- 1 medium yellow onion, thinly sliced
- 2 medium zucchini, sliced thin
- 2 yellow (summer) squashes, sliced thin
- 2 tablespoons chicken stock
- salt
- black pepper

Combine all ingredients in the crock of a slow cooker. Set the slow cooker to low and cook for about 2 hours.

White Sweet Potato Casserole

- 6 white sweet potatoes, peeled and chopped into bite size uniform pieces
- 1 large **white** onion
- ¼ cup diced celery
- 3 tablespoons cornstarch
- 3 cups chicken broth
- 4 tablespoons yellow prepared mustard
- 1 teaspoon salt
- 2 tablespoons black pepper
- 4 tablespoons melted dairy free butter or oil

In a skillet melt the butter or heat the oil, add the cornstarch and using a whisk, combine well into a roux.
Add chicken broth and continue to whisk until a thick sauce. Add more broth in order to get to the consistency you prefer.
Add the yellow prepared mustard. Taste and add salt and pepper to your taste.

Chop the potatoes, onions, and the celery and place in the slow cooker. Add the sauce.
Cook on high about 3-4 hours or low about 5 until the potatoes are tender.

I find white sweet potatoes VERY sweet so you need the mustard to balance that sweetness.

Whole Cauliflower

- 1 whole Cauliflower
- 3 Tbsp Oil
- 1 cup chicken broth
- 5 Tbsp ground mustard
- 2 garlic cloves, smashed and minced
- 2 Tbsp Oregano
- 2 Tbsp Parsley
- Salt & Pepper

Cut the stem and green leaves from the bottom of the cauliflower. Trim the cauliflower head up just enough to allow it to sit flat.

Rub the cauliflower with the oil or you could use melted non-dairy butter.

In a small bowl combine all of the spices: ground mustard, oregano, parsley, salt and pepper. If you would normally add paprika instead add 1/2 teaspoon cumin. If you do not have ground mustard try using lemon pepper instead.

Rub the cauliflower all over the top with the spice mix.

Spread the minced garlic over the head of cauliflower.

Wrap the cauliflower with a large piece of foil making sure to seal it well. Please note that you will need to open the top to add the broth later in the cooking time.

Cook in the slow cooker on high for four hours.

After 4 hours open the foil and pour on the broth. Then cook for another hour on high.

Remove the cauliflower to a serving bowl. Using a fork, separate.

The cauliflower should be quite soft and almost creamy.

SUPPORTING INGREDIENTS

All nuts and seeds are okay.
Avoid soy nuts which are actually soy beans.

Eggs are gluten free, soy free, dairy free and nightshade free.

The most commonly used seasonings that are gluten free, dairy free, soy free and nightshade free:

(avoid spice mixes and seasoning packets)

Basil	Onion powder
Bay leaves	Oregano
Black pepper	Rosemary
Cinnamon	Sage
Cumin	Salt
Garlic	Tarragon
Ginger	Thyme
Nutmeg	Turmeric

Avoid these nightshades: cayenne, chili powder,
Paprika and red pepper

Gluten Free Tortillas: Hard to find in all parts of the country but when you do be sure to heat the tortilla briefly on each side in a hot, dry skillet. Gluten free tortillas simply cannot be eaten as you would any other tortilla without that quick hot stove-top heating.

During the summer months I prefer to use iceberg lettuce as a vessel whenever possible.

Nightshade Free Taco Seasoning:

- 4 tablespoons cumin
- 3 tablespoons oregano
- 2 tablespoon sea salt
- 2 tablespoon black pepper
- 2 tablespoon coriander
- 2 tablespoon onion powder
- 1 tablespoon cornstarch

Combine these ingredients first in their own bowl or jar. Combine well.
Add to one can of pureed canned carrots (with the liquid) and 1 tablespoon Worcestershire Sauce (GF). Add this to 2 pounds of ground beef that has been browned.
Half the amount of spices and pureed carrots if using just one pound of ground beef.
Allow to simmer about 20 minutes uncovered.

Watermelon is an excellent substitute for tomatoes when making salsa. Dice the watermelon and combine with fresh cilantro, diced onion, oil, lime juice, salt and pepper. Add garlic if you normally add garlic to your salsa!

Avoid Soybean oil which is sometimes used in oil blends and it is the ingredient of Vegetable Oil.

Pork Seasoning

Prepared Italian sausage and prepared breakfast sausage may have nightshades. Easily make it yourself by purchasing ground pork (in the Styrofoam tray) in the meat department and add the following seasonings:

For Italian sausage:

- 1 teaspoon salt
- 1 tablespoon Italian seasoning
- ½ teaspoon fennel
- ½ teaspoon garlic
- ½ teaspoon black pepper (more to taste)
- 1 tablespoon oil

You could optionally add oregano or basil for a stronger profile that you prefer.

Combine well and use as you normally would.

For breakfast sausage:

- 1 teaspoon salt
- 1 teaspoon black pepper
- 1 tablespoon sage
- ½ teaspoon cumin
- ¼ teaspoon thyme
- ¼ teaspoon oregano
- 1 teaspoon brown sugar or honey (optional)
- 1 tablespoon oil

Combine well and use as you normally would. The only time I like to add the honey is when I am in the mood to add more black pepper for a sausage that delivers a higher heat level. Otherwise, I generally leave out the honey.

* * *

We thank you for going back to Amazon and leaving your own review for this book.

Paula Henderson's Amazon Authors Page:
amazon.com/author/paulachenderson

Check out the authors other gluten free, dairy free, soy free, and nightshade free cookbooks:

1. Simple Gluten Free, Dairy Free, Soy Free, and Nightshade Free Holiday Recipes: Familiar Menu Ideas with recipes your family will know and love : https://amzn.to/35smxeP
2. A Comprehensive Gluten & Dairy Free Grocery List: Over 1000 Food Items From Every Department: https://amzn.to/2D1jSgf
3. Gluten and Dairy Free Living Recipes: https://amzn.to/2XENw4f
4. Lettuce Amaze You: 100% Dairy, Gluten, Soy, Nightshade and Grain Free Lettuce Recipes: https://amzn.to/2D3Pp19
5. A Gluten And Dairy Free, Grain Free, Soy Free, And Nightshade Free Grocery List: https://amzn.to/2QCv2jk

#CommissionsEarned

Made in the USA
Las Vegas, NV
18 April 2023